Understanding
MIFEPRISTONE

A Comprehensive Guide to Medical Use, Benefits, and Ethical Considerations

Mehmet Bayram

PUBLISHED BY:
Mehmet Bayram

884 Nelson Mandela Drive,
Bochum, Limpopo. South Africa.

Title | Understanding MIFEPRISTONE
Author | Mehmet Bayram
First Print | 2024

Self-Publishing Titans
www.selfpublishingtitans.com
Made by human

Table of Contents

Mifepristone: An Introduction

Overview

Mifepristone, also known by its initial developmental code name RU-486, is a medication typically used in combination with another drug called misoprostol to induce abortion during the early stages of pregnancy. It is also used in the treatment of high blood sugar levels in adults with Cushing's syndrome and has applications in certain cancers and as an emergency contraceptive.

Mechanism of Action

Mifepristone is a synthetic steroid that functions primarily as a progesterone receptor antagonist. By blocking the action of progesterone, a hormone crucial for the continuation of pregnancy, mifepristone causes the lining of the uterus to thin and prevents the embryo from staying implanted. This disruption facilitates the subsequent expulsion of the embryo when followed by the administration of misoprostol.

Usage

- Medical Abortion: When used for abortion, mifepristone is typically given in a single dose, followed by misoprostol 24 to 48 hours later to induce uterine contractions and expel the pregnancy.

- Cushing's Syndrome: For patients with Cushing's syndrome, mifepristone helps manage hyperglycemia due to high cortisol levels.

- Emergency Contraception and Cancer Treatment: Although less common, mifepristone's ability to block progesterone makes it useful in these areas.

Discovery and Development

Mifepristone was developed by the French pharmaceutical company Roussel Uclaf in 1980. The compound was synthesized by chemist Georges Teutsch, and its potential as an abortifacient was recognized soon after. Early clinical trials demonstrated its efficacy and safety, leading to its approval in France in 1988.

Controversies and Approval

The development and distribution of mifepristone have been fraught with political and ethical controversies, particularly in the United States. After its approval in France, there was significant international interest but also substantial opposition, particularly from anti-abortion groups. Despite the controversies, the drug was eventually approved by the U.S. Food and Drug Administration (FDA) in 2000, under stringent regulations.

Global Impact

Since its introduction, mifepristone has become an integral part of medical abortion practices worldwide. It is included in the World

Health Organization's List of Essential Medicines, which underscores its importance in modern healthcare.

Ongoing Research

Research into mifepristone continues, with studies exploring its potential uses beyond abortion and Cushing's syndrome. These include its effectiveness in treating various cancers, fibroids, endometriosis, and its potential neuroprotective effects.

Mifepristone's development journey highlights the intersection of science, medicine, politics, and ethics, reflecting its complex role in society today.

Pharmacology of Mifepristone

Mechanism of Action

Mifepristone primarily acts as a competitive antagonist at progesterone receptors. Progesterone is a hormone critical for the maintenance of pregnancy. By blocking progesterone receptors, mifepristone prevents the hormone from exerting its effects on the uterine lining (endometrium), leading to the following actions:

- Decidual Breakdown: The drug induces changes in the endometrial lining, causing it to break down and detach. This prevents the embryo from continuing to develop and maintaining implantation.

- Cervical Softening and Dilation: Mifepristone softens the cervix, making it easier for the subsequent expulsion of the pregnancy.

- Increased Uterine Contractility: Although primarily mediated by the subsequent administration of misoprostol, mifepristone increases the sensitivity of the uterus to prostaglandins, leading to stronger uterine contractions that help expel the pregnancy.

Pharmacokinetics

- Absorption: Mifepristone is well absorbed after oral administration. The peak plasma concentration is typically reached within 1-2 hours.

- Distribution: Mifepristone is highly protein-bound, mainly to albumin and alpha-1-acid glycoprotein. Its large volume of distribution suggests extensive tissue distribution.

- Metabolism: The drug is metabolized primarily by the liver via cytochrome P450 3A4 (CYP3A4) enzymes. It undergoes demethylation and hydroxylation to form its active metabolites.

- Elimination: Mifepristone and its metabolites are excreted primarily through feces, with a small amount eliminated via urine. The elimination half-life is approximately 18-25 hours, but this can be longer due to the drug's extensive tissue binding.

Pharmacodynamics

- Receptor Binding: Mifepristone binds to the progesterone receptor with a higher affinity than progesterone itself, effectively blocking its action. This leads to the detachment of the embryo and changes in the uterine lining.

- Prostaglandin Sensitization: By blocking progesterone, mifepristone increases the uterus's sensitivity to prostaglandins (e.g., misoprostol), which are necessary for inducing uterine contractions and completing the abortion process.

- Glucocorticoid Receptor Antagonism: At higher doses, mifepristone also acts as a glucocorticoid receptor antagonist. This property is exploited in the treatment of Cushing's syndrome, where the drug helps reduce the effects of excess cortisol.

- Anti-Proliferative Effects: Mifepristone exhibits anti-proliferative effects on endometrial and certain cancer cells, which is being explored for therapeutic applications beyond its use in reproductive health.

Clinical Implications

- Medical Abortion: The combination of mifepristone and misoprostol is highly effective for early medical abortion, with success rates exceeding 95% when used within the first 10 weeks of pregnancy.

- Cushing's Syndrome: In patients with endogenous

Cushing's syndrome, mifepristone helps control hyperglycemia secondary to hypercortisolism.

- Potential Therapeutic Uses: Research is ongoing to explore the use of mifepristone in treating other conditions like uterine fibroids, endometriosis, certain types of cancer, and as an emergency contraceptive due to its ability to inhibit ovulation and alter the endometrial lining.

Mifepristone's pharmacological profile

underscores its diverse therapeutic potential, driven by its ability to modulate hormone receptors critical to various physiological processes.

Medical Uses of Mifepristone

Indications

1. Medical Abortion:

- Used in combination with misoprostol for the termination of early pregnancy (up to 10 weeks gestation).

2. Cushing's Syndrome:

- For the control of hyperglycemia secondary to hypercortisolism in adults with endogenous Cushing's syndrome who have type 2 diabetes mellitus or glucose intolerance and have not responded to surgical treatment or are not candidates for surgery.

3. Emergency Contraception:

- Although not a primary indication, mifepristone can be used off-label as an emergency contraceptive to prevent pregnancy after unprotected sex or contraceptive failure.

4. Other Potential Uses:

- Research is ongoing into the use of mifepristone for treating uterine fibroids, endometriosis, certain types of cancer (e.g., breast cancer, meningioma), and as a part of hormone therapy.

Dosage and Administration

1. Medical Abortion:

- Up to 10 Weeks Gestation:

- Mifepristone: 200 mg orally as a single dose.

- Misoprostol: 800 mcg (four 200 mcg tablets) buccally, sublingually, or vaginally 24 to 48 hours after taking mifepristone.

2. Cushing's Syndrome:

- Starting Dose: 300 mg orally once daily.

- The dose may be increased in 300 mg increments based on clinical response and tolerability, up to a maximum of 1200 mg once daily.

3. Emergency Contraception (Off-Label):

- Dosage: 10-25 mg orally within 72 hours of unprotected intercourse.

Efficacy

1. Medical Abortion:

- Effectiveness: The combination of mifepristone and misoprostol is highly effective, with success rates exceeding 95% for pregnancies up to 10 weeks gestation.

- Safety: The regimen is generally safe when used as directed, with most complications being mild and manageable (e.g., bleeding, cramping).

2. Cushing's Syndrome:

- Effectiveness: Mifepristone is effective in controlling hyperglycemia secondary to hypercortisolism, leading to significant improvements in glucose levels and clinical symptoms.

- Safety: Common side effects include fatigue, nausea, headache, and hypokalemia. Monitoring is necessary to manage potential adverse effects.

3. Emergency Contraception:

- Effectiveness: When used off-label as emergency contraception, mifepristone has shown efficacy comparable to other emergency contraceptives, with a high success rate in preventing pregnancy when taken within 72 hours of unprotected intercourse.

Mifepristone is a versatile medication with proven efficacy in medical abortion and managing hyperglycemia in Cushing's syndrome. Its potential uses in emergency contraception and other medical conditions are under investigation, reflecting its broad therapeutic potential. Proper dosage and administration are crucial to achieving optimal outcomes and minimizing side effects.

Safety and Side Effects of Mifepristone

Common Side Effects

1. Gastrointestinal Symptoms:

   - Nausea

   - Vomiting

   - Diarrhea

   - Abdominal pain and cramping

2. General Symptoms:

   - Fatigue

   - Dizziness

- Headache

3. Reproductive System:

- Heavy bleeding or spotting

- Uterine cramping

- Pelvic pain

4. Other:

- Chills or fever (typically associated with misoprostol use)

Serious Adverse Effects

1. Severe Bleeding:

- Heavy and prolonged bleeding requiring medical

intervention, including transfusion in rare cases.

2. Infection:

- Rare cases of serious infection, including sepsis, have been reported after medical abortion.

- Signs include fever, severe abdominal pain, or prolonged malaise.

3. Incomplete Abortion:

- Failure to completely expel the pregnancy tissue, necessitating surgical intervention.

4. Cardiovascular Effects:

- Hypotension or hypertension

- Arrhythmias, especially in patients with preexisting conditions

Contraindications

1. Pregnancy Exceeding 10 Weeks Gestation:

- Mifepristone is not recommended for termination of pregnancies beyond 10 weeks.

2. Ectopic Pregnancy:

- Mifepristone is ineffective for ectopic pregnancies and may pose serious health risks.

3. Chronic Adrenal Failure:

- Due to its anti-glucocorticoid effects, mifepristone is contraindicated in patients with adrenal insufficiency.

4. Hemorrhagic Disorders:

- Patients with coagulation disorders or those on anticoagulant therapy are at higher risk of severe bleeding.

5. Allergy to Mifepristone or Misoprostol:

- Hypersensitivity to the drug or any component of the formulation.

6. Inherited Porphyria:

- Mifepristone is contraindicated in patients with inherited porphyria.

Interactions with Other Medications

1. CYP3A4 Inhibitors:

- Drugs like ketoconazole, itraconazole, and

erythromycin can increase mifepristone levels, potentially leading to adverse effects.

2. CYP3A4 Inducers:

- Rifampin, phenytoin, and St. John's wort may decrease mifepristone levels, reducing its efficacy.

3. Corticosteroids:

- Concomitant use can reduce the effectiveness of corticosteroids due to mifepristone's glucocorticoid receptor antagonism.

4. Anticoagulants:

- Increased risk of bleeding when used with anticoagulants like warfarin or antiplatelet agents.

5. Nonsteroidal Anti-Inflammatory Drugs (NSAIDs):

- Potential to diminish the efficacy of mifepristone by counteracting prostaglandin-induced uterine contractions.

While mifepristone is generally safe and effective

when used as directed, it is important to be aware of its common side effects and potential serious adverse effects. Proper patient selection, adherence to contraindications, and monitoring for interactions with other medications are crucial to ensure patient safety and achieve optimal therapeutic outcomes.

Clinical Guidelines for Mifepristone

Protocols for Medical Abortion

Up to 10 Weeks Gestation:

1. Initial Visit:

-   Confirm intrauterine pregnancy via ultrasound.

-   Review medical history and assess for contraindications.

-   Provide counseling on the procedure, potential side

effects, and follow-up requirements.

2. Administration:

- Day 1: Mifepristone 200 mg orally as a single dose.

- Day 2-3: Misoprostol 800 mcg (four 200 mcg tablets) buccally, sublingually, or vaginally 24 to 48 hours after taking mifepristone.

- Alternative Regimens: May include additional doses of misoprostol if the initial dose is not effective.

3. Follow-Up:

- Clinical evaluation or ultrasound 7-14 days after administration to confirm complete expulsion of pregnancy.

- If incomplete abortion is suspected, additional misoprostol or surgical intervention may be required.

Use in Different Trimesters

First Trimester (Up to 10 Weeks):

- The standard regimen of mifepristone followed by misoprostol is used.

- High efficacy with a low rate of complications.

Second Trimester (11-24 Weeks):

- Medical abortion beyond 10 weeks typically involves higher doses and additional doses of misoprostol.

- Protocols may vary based on local regulations and clinical guidelines.

Beyond 24 Weeks:

- Mifepristone is rarely used for elective abortions beyond

24 weeks due to legal, ethical, and medical considerations.

- Indications may include severe fetal anomalies or significant maternal health risks.

- Administration should be done in specialized medical settings with appropriate monitoring and support.

Post-Administration Care

1. Monitoring:

- Patients should be monitored for signs of

excessive bleeding, infection, and incomplete abortion.

- Emergency contact information should be provided for any complications.

2. Pain Management:

- NSAIDs like ibuprofen can be used to manage cramping and pain.

- Avoid aspirin due to the risk of increased bleeding.

3. Counseling and Support:

- Provide emotional support and counseling before and after the procedure.

- Discuss contraceptive options to prevent future unintended pregnancies.

4. Follow-Up Visit:

- A follow-up visit 7-14 days post-administration to ensure the abortion is complete.

- An ultrasound or clinical examination may be performed to confirm.

5. Signs of Complications:

- Patients should be educated on signs of potential complications, such as heavy bleeding (soaking more than two pads per hour for two consecutive hours), severe abdominal pain not relieved by pain medication, fever, or foul-smelling discharge.

- Immediate medical attention should be sought if any of these symptoms occur.

Mifepristone, in combination with misoprostol, is a highly effective regimen for medical abortion, primarily used within the first 10 weeks of pregnancy. Protocols vary for different trimesters, and comprehensive post-administration care is essential to ensure patient safety and the complete expulsion of the pregnancy. Proper patient selection, adherence to guidelines, and providing adequate support and follow-up care are crucial for optimal outcomes.

Regulatory Status of Mifepristone

Approval by Health Authorities

1. United States:

- Approved by the U.S. Food and Drug Administration (FDA) in 2000 for medical abortion up to 10 weeks gestation.

- Also approved for the management of hyperglycemia secondary to hypercortisolism in Cushing's syndrome.

2. European Union:

- Approved by the European Medicines Agency (EMA) for medical abortion up to 10 weeks gestation and for use in combination with misoprostol.

3. World Health Organization (WHO):

- Included in the WHO Model List of Essential Medicines, highlighting its importance in reproductive health.

4. Other Countries:

- Approved in numerous countries worldwide, including Canada, Australia, New Zealand, and many countries in Asia, Africa, and Latin America, with varying indications and usage guidelines.

Variations by Country

1.   Availability and Restrictions:

- United States: Access is regulated, with mifepristone available through certified healthcare providers and pharmacies under the FDA's

Risk Evaluation and Mitigation Strategy (REMS) program.

- France: First country to approve mifepristone (1988); available through healthcare providers.

- United Kingdom: Available through the National Health Service (NHS) and private clinics.

- China and India: Widely available and used for medical abortion, with varying degrees of regulation.

- Ireland: Legalized in 2018 following a referendum, with

mifepristone available under specific guidelines.

2. Legal Status:

- In some countries, mifepristone is strictly regulated or banned due to legal and ethical considerations surrounding abortion.

- Access and use may vary significantly, even within regions of the same country, based on local laws and regulations.

Legal and Ethical Considerations

1. Abortion Laws:

   - Permissive: Countries like Canada, most of Western Europe, and parts of Latin America have relatively liberal abortion laws, allowing the use of mifepristone.

   - Restrictive: Countries in regions like Africa, Southeast Asia, and the Middle East often have more restrictive laws, limiting or prohibiting access to mifepristone.

- Variable: In countries like the United States, access can vary widely by state, with some states imposing significant restrictions.

2. Ethical Debates:

- Pro-Choice vs. Pro-Life: The use of mifepristone for medical abortion is a central issue in the broader pro-choice versus pro-life debate.

- Women's Rights: Advocates argue that access to mifepristone is essential for women's reproductive rights and health.

- Fetal Rights: Opponents often focus on the moral and ethical considerations regarding the rights of the fetus.

3. Healthcare Provider Conscience:

- Some countries have provisions allowing healthcare providers to refuse to prescribe or administer mifepristone based on personal or religious beliefs.

- Balancing provider conscience rights with patient

access remains a contentious issue.

4. Cultural and Religious Influences:

- Cultural norms and religious beliefs significantly influence the acceptance and use of mifepristone.

- In some regions, cultural stigmas around abortion can limit access despite legal approval.

The regulatory status of mifepristone varies widely across the globe, reflecting differing legal, ethical, and cultural attitudes toward abortion and reproductive health. While many countries have approved its use for medical abortion and other indications, access and availability are often subject to significant restrictions and regulations. The legal and ethical considerations surrounding mifepristone continue to shape its global landscape, highlighting the complex interplay between health policy, societal values, and individual rights.

Research and Development of Mifepristone

Ongoing Clinical Trials

1. Cancer Treatment:

- Breast Cancer: Investigating mifepristone's potential role in hormone receptor-positive breast cancer as a combination therapy with other treatments.

- Meningioma: Exploring its use in treating meningiomas, particularly those expressing progesterone receptors.

2. Uterine Fibroids and Endometriosis:

- Assessing mifepristone's efficacy in reducing symptoms and size of uterine fibroids and managing pain associated with endometriosis.

3. Emergency Contraception:

- Studies evaluating its effectiveness and safety as an emergency contraceptive option, particularly in comparison to other methods.

4. Neurological Disorders:

- Research into potential neuroprotective effects in conditions like Alzheimer's disease and traumatic brain injury.

Recent Findings

1. Breast Cancer: Recent studies suggest that mifepristone, when combined with other therapies, may help overcome resistance to hormone therapy in certain breast cancer subtypes.

2. Cushing's Syndrome: Continued research focuses on optimizing dosing and

long-term outcomes in managing hypercortisolism and associated metabolic complications.

3. Medical Abortion: Advances in administration protocols and follow-up care have improved efficacy and safety profiles, with ongoing efforts to streamline procedures and reduce complications.

4. Psychiatric Disorders: Studies exploring mifepristone's potential in treating psychiatric conditions such as depression and bipolar disorder through

modulation of glucocorticoid receptors.

Future Directions

1. Precision Medicine Approaches: Tailoring mifepristone therapy based on genetic profiles and tumor characteristics to optimize treatment outcomes in cancer and other conditions.

2. Combination Therapies: Investigating synergistic effects of mifepristone with other drugs or therapies to enhance efficacy and reduce side effects.

3. Expanded Indications: Exploring new applications beyond current approved uses, potentially including autoimmune disorders, infertility treatments, and other hormone-related conditions.

4. Safety and Tolerability: Continual research into minimizing adverse effects and improving patient tolerance through modified formulations or delivery methods.

Mifepristone continues to be a subject of active research and development across various medical fields. Ongoing clinical trials explore its potential in cancer treatment, gynecological disorders, emergency contraception, and neurological conditions. Recent findings highlight promising outcomes in breast cancer therapy and expanding understanding of its mechanisms in hormonal regulation and disease management. Future directions aim to advance precision medicine approaches, explore new therapeutic avenues, and enhance safety profiles, underscoring its evolving role in modern healthcare.

Patient Information on Mifepristone

Counseling and Education

1. Procedure Explanation:

- Explain the medical abortion procedure, including the use of mifepristone and misoprostol, the expected timeline, and what to expect during and after the process.

2. Side Effects and Risks:

- Discuss common side effects such as nausea, cramping, and bleeding, as well as potential serious risks like heavy bleeding, infection, and incomplete abortion.

3. Follow-Up Care:

- Emphasize the importance of attending follow-up appointments to confirm the completion of the abortion and address any concerns or complications.

4. Contraception Counseling:

- Provide information on contraceptive options to prevent future unintended pregnancies, including discussing the timing and effectiveness of different methods.

5. Emotional Support:

- Offer emotional support and resources for coping with the decision and any emotional responses that may arise during or after the procedure.

Support Resources

1. Healthcare Providers:

- Encourage patients to ask questions and seek clarification from their healthcare provider regarding any aspect of the procedure or their health concerns.

2. Hotlines and Helplines:

- Provide contact information for hotlines or helplines that offer confidential counseling and support for patients considering or undergoing medical abortion.

3. Patient Advocacy Groups:

- Refer patients to reputable organizations or advocacy groups that provide information, support, and advocacy for reproductive health and rights.

4. Online Resources:

- Recommend trusted websites and online forums where patients can access accurate information, share experiences, and connect with others who have undergone similar procedures.

Frequently Asked Questions

1. How does mifepristone work?

- Explain that mifepristone blocks progesterone receptors, causing the uterus lining to break down and the pregnancy to end.

2. What are the side effects?

- Outline common side effects like nausea, cramping, and bleeding, and mention rare but serious risks such as heavy bleeding and infection.

3. How effective is medical abortion with mifepristone?

- Provide statistics on the high effectiveness of medical abortion when used within the recommended timeframe (up to 10 weeks gestation).

4. What should I do if I experience severe symptoms?

- Instruct patients to seek medical attention immediately if they experience severe bleeding, intense pain, fever, or other concerning symptoms.

5. Will medical abortion affect my future fertility?

- Assure patients that medical abortion with mifepristone has not been shown to affect future fertility or increase the risk of complications in future pregnancies.

Patient counseling and education are crucial aspects of mifepristone administration for medical abortion. Providing comprehensive information on the procedure, side effects, follow-up care, contraception options, and emotional support helps patients make informed decisions and manage their health effectively. Access to support resources, including healthcare providers, hotlines, advocacy groups, and online information, enhances patient support and ensures they receive necessary care and guidance throughout the process.

Controversies and Debates Surrounding Mifepristone

Political and Social Context

1. Abortion Rights:

- Mifepristone's availability and use are central to debates over abortion rights and reproductive autonomy.

- In countries with varying legal frameworks, political positions often influence access and availability, impacting healthcare policy and public health outcomes.

2. Legislative Actions:

- Political debates and legislative actions can lead to changes in regulations affecting mifepristone's accessibility, including restrictions on its use and distribution.

3. Public Opinion:

- Views on abortion and mifepristone vary widely across societies, influenced by cultural, religious, and ethical beliefs.

- Public discourse often reflects diverse perspectives,

shaping public policy and healthcare practices.

Ethical Discussions

1. Fetal Rights vs. Women's Rights:

   - Ethical debates center on balancing the rights of the fetus with the rights of women to control their reproductive health.

   - Perspectives vary on when personhood begins and the ethical implications of terminating pregnancies using mifepristone.

2.   Healthcare   Provider
Conscience:

- Issues arise regarding
healthcare providers' rights to
conscientious   objection,
potentially   limiting   patient
access to mifepristone and
related services.

3. Informed Consent:

- Ensuring informed consent
involves   providing
comprehensive information on
mifepristone's risks, benefits,
and alternatives, reflecting
ethical principles of autonomy
and patient decision-making.

Impact on Healthcare Access

1. Geographical Disparities:

- Access to mifepristone varies geographically, influenced by local laws, healthcare infrastructure, and provider availability.

- Rural and underserved areas may face greater challenges in accessing mifepristone and comprehensive reproductive healthcare services.

2. Stigma and Barriers:

- Stigma surrounding abortion and mifepristone use can create barriers to access, affecting patient willingness to seek care and healthcare provider willingness to offer services.

3. Legal and Regulatory Challenges:

- Legal restrictions and regulatory hurdles, such as mandatory waiting periods or physician requirements, can impede timely access to mifepristone and medical abortion services.

Mifepristone's controversies and debates intersect political, social, and ethical dimensions, shaping healthcare access and policy worldwide. Political and legislative actions, ethical considerations regarding women's rights and fetal rights, and healthcare provider conscience rights contribute to complex discussions surrounding mifepristone's use. These debates impact healthcare access, influencing patient care, provider practices, and public health outcomes, highlighting the ongoing challenges and implications in reproductive healthcare policy and practice.

THE END